I0470589

MedicalCenter.com

The Key Facts on Medicare

<u>Everything You Need to Know About Medicare</u>

-Usable Medical Information for the Patient-

By Patrick W. Nee

www.MedicalCenter.com

Published by:

MedicalCenter.com

96 Walter Street/ Suite 200

Boston, MA 02131, USA

Tel: 617-354-7722

www.MedicalCenter.com

manager@medicalcenter.com

Table of Contents

Chapter 1: Basic Information

What Is Medicare?

Medicare is a federal health insurance program for people

- age 65 and older
- under age 65 with certain disabilities who have been receiving Social Security disability benefits for a certain amount of time (24 months in most cases)
- of any age who have End-Stage Renal Disease (ESRD), which is permanent kidney failure requiring dialysis or a transplant.

Medicare helps with the cost of health care, but it does not cover all medical expenses.

The Basics

Medicare Has Four Parts

- Part A - Hospital insurance
- Part B - Medical insurance

- Part C - Medicare Advantage Plans like HMOs (health maintenance organizations) and PPOs (preferred provider organizations)
- Part D - Medicare prescription drug coverage

Medicare Part A helps cover inpatient care in hospitals. Part A also helps cover skilled nursing facility care, hospice care, and home health care, under certain conditions.

Medicare Part B helps cover medical services such as doctor's services, outpatient care, and other medical services that Part A doesn't cover. Part B also covers some preventive services, such as flu shots and diabetes screening, to help people maintain their health and to keep certain illnesses from getting worse.

Medicare Advantage Plans, sometimes known as Medicare Part C, are health plans people can join to get their Medicare benefits. These plans cover hospital costs (Part A), medical costs (Part B), and sometimes prescription drug costs (Part D). Medicare Advantage Plans may also offer extra coverage, such as vision, hearing, dental, and/or health and wellness programs. Medicare Advantage Plans are managed by private insurance companies approved by Medicare.

Medicare Part D helps pay for medications that a doctor may prescribe. This coverage may help lower prescription drug costs. These plans are run by insurance companies and other private companies approved by Medicare.

What Medicare Doesn't Cover

Medicare doesn't cover everything. For example, Medicare doesn't cover cosmetic surgery, health care you get while traveling outside of the United States (except in limited cases), hearing aids, most hearing exams, long-term care (like care in a nursing home), most eyeglasses, most dental care and dentures, and more. Some of these services may be covered by a Medicare Advantage Plan.

Medicaid

Some people think that Medicare and Medicaid are the same, but they are two different programs. Medicaid is a state-run program that provides hospital and medical coverage for people with low income and little or no resources. Each state has its own rules about who is eligible and what is covered under Medicaid. Some people qualify for both Medicare and Medicaid.

If you have questions about Medicaid, you can call your State Medical Assistance (Medicaid) office for more information.

Chapter 2: Medicare Health Plans

Medicare gives you choices in how you get your health and prescription drug coverage. A person can choose Original Medicare, one of the Medicare Advantage Plans, or other Medicare plans.

Original Medicare

Original Medicare is managed by the Federal government and lets people with Medicare go to any doctor, hospital, or other health care provider who accepts Medicare. It is a fee-for-service plan, meaning that the person with Medicare usually pays a fee for each service. Medicare pays its share of an approved amount up to certain limits, and the person with Medicare pays the rest.

People in Original Medicare must choose and join a Medicare Prescription Drug Plan if they want to get Medicare prescription drug coverage.

Medicare Advantage Plans

Medicare Advantage Plans are health plans approved by Medicare and run by private companies. They are part of the Medicare program, and are sometimes called "Part C."

Medicare Advantage Plans are available in many areas of the country, and a person who joins one of these plans

- is still in the Medicare program
- still has Medicare rights and protections
- still gets all regular Medicare-covered services offered under Part A and Part B.
- may get additional benefits offered through the plan, including Medicare prescription drug coverage. Other extra benefits could include coverage for vision, hearing, or dental care, and/or health and wellness program.

Medicare Advantage Plans include Medicare Health Maintenance Organization (HMO) Plans, Medicare

Preferred Provider Organization (PPO) Plans, Medicare Private Fee-for-Service (PFFS) Plans, Medicare Special Needs Plans (SNPs), and Medicare Medical Savings Accounts (MSAs). In most of these plans, there are generally extra benefits and lower co-payments than in Original Medicare. However, a person may have to see doctors that belong to the plan or go to certain hospitals to get services. A person can switch plans each year in the fall, if desired.

How to Join

To join a Medicare Advantage Plan, a person must

- live in the plan's geographic service area or continuation area
- not have End-Stage Renal Disease (ESRD)
- have Medicare Part A and Part B
- pay the monthly Medicare Part B premium to Medicare. In addition, it might be necessary to pay a monthly premium to the

Medicare Advantage Plan for the extra benefits that they offer.

When to Join

People can join a Medicare Advantage Plan when they first become eligible for Medicare. They can switch to another Medicare Advantage Plan or to Original Medicare during the Annual Election Period from October 15 - December 7. A person can only belong to one Medicare Advantage program at a time, and enrollment in a plan is generally for a calendar year.

Switching to Original Medicare

Between January 1 through February 14, a person can leave an MA plan and switch to Original Medicare. If the person makes this change, he or she may also join a Medicare Prescription Drug Plan to add drug coverage. Coverage begins the first of the month after the plan receives the enrollment form.

For More Information

To find out what Medicare Advantage Plans are available in your area, visit**http://www.medicare.gov** and choose the link Compare Health Plans and Medigap Policies in Your Area to use the Medicare Options Compare tool, or call 1-800-MEDICARE (1-800-633-4227).

Medigap

People who choose Original Medicare may want to consider Medigap, a type of Medicare supplement insurance. Medigap policies are sold by private insurance companies to fill gaps in Original Medicare Plan coverage, such as out-of-pocket costs for Medicare co-insurance and deductibles, or for services not covered by Medicare. A Medigap policy only works with Original Medicare. A person who joins a Medicare Advantage Plan generally doesn't need (and can't use) a Medigap policy.

The PACE Program

Programs of All-Inclusive Care for the Elderly (PACE)

Other plans include Medicare Cost Plans and Programs of All-Inclusive Care for the Elderly (PACE). PACE combines medical, social, and long-term care services, and prescription drug coverage for frail, elderly people who get health care in the community.

To qualify for PACE, people must be at least age 55, live in the PACE service area, meet their state's standard for nursing home level care, and be able to live safely in a community setting at the time of enrollment. Call the State Medical Assistance (Medicaid) office or visit **http://www.cms.hhs.gov/pace** to find out about eligibility and to see if there is a PACE site nearby.

Help in Choosing a Plan

To get help choosing a Medicare health plan, call 1-800-Medicare (1-800-633-4227). TTY users should call 1-877-486-2048. To compare health plan choices in your area, visit **www.medicare.gov**, or go to the Medicare Plan Finder at **www.medicare.gov/find-a-plan/questions/home.aspx**.

Chapter 3: Getting Medicare

Enrollment is Automatic for Many

Enrollment in Medicare is automatic for a person who is turning 65 and who is already getting Social Security benefits, or who will start getting them at age 65. A Medicare card will be mailed out about three months before the 65th birthday. If a person isn't getting Social Security benefits when he or she turns age 65, the person will have to sign up for Medicare.

Automatic enrollment includes Part A and Part B. If people don't want Part B, they should follow the instructions that come with the card, and send the card back. If they keep the card, they keep Part B. Enrollment is also automatic for a person who has been entitled to Social Security disability benefits for at least 24 months. A Medicare card is mailed out about 3 months before the 25th month of disability benefits.

A person with amyotrophic lateral sclerosis (also known as Lou Gehrig's disease) will get a Medicare card about 4 weeks after qualifying for Medicare. A person with end-stage renal disease, or ESRD, does not need to be receiving Social Security disability benefits to qualify for Medicare, and may still be working.

Which Agencies Handle Enrollment?

The Centers for Medicare and Medicaid Services (CMS) administers Medicare, but the Social Security Administration (SSA) is responsible for enrolling most people in Medicare. The Railroad Retirement board is responsible for enrolling railroad retirees. For questions about Medicare enrollment, or to apply for Medicare benefits, call SSA at 1-800-772-1213, or go to **http://www.ssa.gov** to find out more.

More on Part A and Part B

Most people don't have to pay a monthly fee, or premium, for Medicare Part A (hospital insurance) when they turn age 65 because they or a spouse paid Medicare taxes while they were working. Enrollment in Medicare Part B (medical insurance) is optional, and most people who choose Part B must pay a monthly premium. Some people with a higher income pay a higher Part B premium. The Social Security Administration will send out a notice if income is above a certain threshold. There may be a late enrollment penalty for Part B if the person doesn't join when he or she is first eligible. People can decide how to get their Medicare benefits. They can choose Original Medicare, one of the Medicare Advantage Plans, or other Medicare health plans.

Plans Vary

Original Medicare and the Medicare Advantage Plans include Part A (hospital insurance) and Part B (medical insurance). However, co-payments and deductibles vary among the different plans. A person who joins Original Medicare, and who wants prescription drug coverage, will need to choose and sign up for a Medicare Prescription Drug plan. A person who joins one of the Medicare Advantage Plans will automatically receive prescription drug coverage through that plan if it is offered, usually for an extra cost. To get help choosing a plan, call 1-800-Medicare (1-800-633-4227). TTY users should call 1-877-486-2048.

If You Have Limited Resources

Your state has programs that pay some or all of the Medicare premiums for people with limited income and resources. Call your state's Medical Assistance (Medicaid) Office to learn about Medicare Savings Programs, or visit **www.medicare.gov**.

Chapter 4: Medicare Basics: Terms to Know

Here is a list of terms providing basic information about Medicare.

Medicare Part A

This is hospital insurance that pays for inpatient hospital stays, care in a skilled nursing facility for a limited period of time, hospice care, and some home health care.

Medicare Part B

This is medical insurance that helps pay for doctor's services, outpatient hospital care, durable medical equipment, and some medical services that aren't covered by Part A.

Medicare Advantage Plan (Part C)

This is a type of Medicare Plan offered by a private company that provides a person with all Medicare Part A and Part B benefits. Also called Part C, Medicare Advantage Plans are HMOs (health maintenance organizations), PPOs (preferred provider organizations), Private Fee-for-Service Plans, and Medical Savings Account Plans. If a person is enrolled in a Medicare Advantage Plan, Medicare services are covered through the plan and aren't paid for under Original Medicare. Some Medicare Advantage Plans offer prescription drug coverage that must follow the same rules as Medicare Prescription Drug Plans. Medicare Advantage Plans may also offer extra coverage, such as vision, hearing, dental, and/or health and wellness programs.

Medicare Prescription Drug Plan (Part D)
This is a stand-alone drug plan, offered by insurers and other private companies to people who get benefits through Original Medicare, a Medicare

Private Fee-for-Service Plan, a Medicare Cost Plan, or a Medicare Medical Savings Account Plan. (Descriptions of these last three plans follow.)

Medicare Health Maintenance Organization (HMO) Plan

This is a type of Medicare Advantage Plan that is available in some areas of the country. Plans must cover all Medicare Part A and Part B health care. Some HMOs cover extra benefits, like extra days in the hospital. In most HMOs, a person can only go to doctors, specialists, or hospitals on the plan's list except in an emergency. The person's costs may be lower than in Original Medicare.

Medicare Preferred Provider Organization (PPO) Plan

This is a type of Medicare Advantage Plan available in a local or regional area in which people pay less if they use doctors, hospitals, and providers that belong to the network. People can use doctors, hospitals, and providers outside of the network for an additional cost. Many Medicare Advantage Plans are PPOs.

Medicare-approved Amount

In Original Medicare, this is the amount a doctor or supplier that accepts assignment can be paid. (Assignment is an agreement between Medicare doctors, health care providers, and suppliers to accept the Medicare-approved amount as payment in full.)

The Medicare-approved amount includes what Medicare pays and any deductible, co-insurance, or co-payment that a patient pays. It may be less than the actual amount a doctor or supplier charges. If a doctor or supplier does accept assignment, Medicare will pay 80 percent of the cost, and the patient pays the rest.

Medicare Cost Plan

A Medicare Cost Plan is a type of HMO, or health maintenance organization. In a Medicare Cost Plan, if people get services outside of the plan's network without a referral, their Medicare-covered services will be paid for under Original Medicare. (The Cost Plan pays for emergency services or urgently needed services.)

Medicare Private Fee-for-Service (PFFS) Plan

This is a type of Medicare Advantage Plan in which people may go to any Medicare-approved doctor or hospital that accepts the plan's payment. The insurance plan, rather than the Medicare Program, decides how much it will pay and what people will pay for the services they get. People may pay more or less for Medicare-covered benefits. They may have extra benefits that Original Medicare doesn't cover.

Medigap Policy

This is Medicare Supplement Insurance sold by private insurance companies to fill "gaps" in Original Medicare Plan coverage.

Medicare Medical Savings Account (MSA) Plan

MSA Plans combine a high-deductible Medicare Advantage Plan like a health maintenance organization (HMO) or preferred provider organization (PPO) with a Medical Savings Account for medical expenses.

Medicare Special Needs Plan

This is a special type of Medicare Advantage Plan that provides more focused and specialized health care for specific groups of people, such as those who have both Medicare and Medicaid, who reside in a nursing home, or have certain chronic medical conditions.

Premium

This is the periodic payment to Medicare, an insurance company, or a health plan for health care or prescription drug coverage.

Chapter 5: Frequently Asked Questions

1. What is Medicare?

Medicare is a federal health insurance program for people

- age 65 and older
- under age 65 with certain disabilities who have been receiving Social Security disability benefits for a certain amount of time (24 months in most cases)
- of any age who have End-Stage Renal Disease (ESRD), which is permanent kidney failure requiring dialysis or a transplant.

Medicare helps with the cost of health care, but it does not cover all medical expenses.

2. What is Medicare Part A and what does it cover?

Medicare Part A is hospital insurance that helps cover inpatient care in hospitals. Part A also helps cover skilled nursing facility care for a limited period of time, hospice care, and home health care, if you meet certain conditions. Most people don't have to pay a monthly premium for Medicare Part A when they turn age 65 because they or a spouse paid Medicare taxes while they were working.

If a person is hospitalized, Medicare helps pay for the following services.

- Care - general nursing
- Room - semiprivate room
- Hospital services - meals, most services and supplies

If a person is hospitalized, Medicare does NOT pay for the following services.

- Care - private-duty nursing
- Room - private room (unless medically necessary)

- Hospital services - television and telephone

3. What is Medicare Part B and what does it cover?

Medicare Part B is medical insurance. It helps cover medical services such as doctor's services, outpatient care and other medical services that Part A doesn't cover. Part B also covers some preventive services, such as flu shots and diabetes screening, to help you maintain your health and to keep certain illnesses from getting worse.

Enrollment in Part B is optional, and most people who choose it must pay a monthly fee, or premium. There may be a late enrollment penalty for Part B if the person doesn't join when he or she is first eligible.

You can also contact your State Health Insurance Assistance Program (SHIP) which gives free health insurance counseling and guidance to people with

Medicare -- or to family and friends who have authorization to help someone with Medicare questions.

To sign up for Medicare Part B, call Social Security at 1-800-772-1213. TTY users should call 1-800-325-0778. If you are getting benefits from the Railroad Retirement Board, call your local RRB office or 1-800-808-0772.

4. What is Medicare Part C and what does it cover?

Medicare Advantage Plans, sometimes known as Medicare Part C, are plans people can join to get their Medicare benefits. Medicare Advantage Plans are available in many areas of the country, and a person who joins one of these plans will get all Medicare-covered benefits. These plans cover hospital costs (Part A), medical costs (Part B), and sometimes prescription drug costs (Part D). Medicare Advantage Plans may also offer extra coverage, such as vision, hearing, dental, and/or health and wellness programs. Medicare Advantage Plans are managed by private insurance companies approved by Medicare.

To join a Medicare Advantage Plan, a person must have Medicare Part A and Part B and must pay the monthly Medicare Part B premium to Medicare. In addition, it might be necessary to pay a monthly premium to the Medicare Advantage Plan for the extra benefits that they offer.

In most of these plans, there are generally extra benefits and lower co-payments than in Original Medicare. (See Question #6 for information about Original Medicare.) However, a person may have to see doctors that belong to the plan or go to certain hospitals to get services. A person can switch plans each year in the fall if desired.

5. What is Medicare Part D and what does it cover?

Medicare Part D helps pay for medications that a doctor may prescribe. This coverage may help lower prescription drug costs.

Medicare drug plans are run by insurance companies and other private companies approved by Medicare. A person who joins Original Medicare and who wants prescription drug coverage will need to choose and sign up for a Medicare Prescription Drug plan (PDP). A person who joins one of the Medicare Advantage Plans will automatically receive prescription drug coverage through that plan if it's offered, usually for an extra cost.

For more information about Medicare Part D, visit **www.medicare.gov**.

6. What is Original Medicare?

Original Medicare is managed by the Federal government and lets people with Medicare go to any doctor, hospital or other health care provider who accepts Medicare. It is a fee-for-service plan, meaning that the person with Medicare usually pays a fee for each service. Medicare pays its share of an approved amount up to certain limits, and the person with Medicare pays the rest.

People in Original Medicare must choose and join a Medicare Prescription Drug Plan if they want to get Medicare prescription drug coverage.

7. What are Medicare Advantage Plans?

Medicare Advantage Plans, sometimes known as Medicare Part C, are plans people can join to get their Medicare benefits. Medicare Advantage Plans are available in many areas of the country, and a person who joins one of these plans will get all Medicare-covered benefits. These plans cover hospital costs (Part A), medical costs (Part B), and sometimes prescription drug costs (Part D). Medicare Advantage Plans may also offer extra coverage, such as vision, hearing, dental, and/or health and wellness programs. Medicare Advantage Plans are managed by private insurance companies approved by Medicare.

To join a Medicare Advantage Plan, a person must have Medicare Part A and Part B and must pay the monthly Medicare Part B premium to Medicare. In addition, it might be necessary to pay a monthly premium to the Medicare Advantage Plan for the extra benefits that they offer.

In most of these plans, there are generally extra benefits and lower co-payments than in Original Medicare. However, a person may have to see doctors that belong to the plan or go to certain hospitals to get services. A person can switch plans each year in the fall if desired.

To get help choosing a plan, call 1-800-Medicare (1-800-633-4227). TTY users should call 1-877-486-2048.

8. How does a person enroll in Medicare?

Enrollment in Medicare is automatic for a person who is turning 65 and who is already getting Social Security benefits, or who will start getting them at age 65. A Medicare card will be mailed out about three months before the 65th birthday. If a person isn't getting Social Security benefits when he or she turns age 65, the person will have to sign up for Medicare.

Automatic enrollment includes Part A and Part B. If people don't want Part B, they should follow the instructions that come with the card, and send the card back. If they keep the card, they keep Part B. Enrollment is also automatic for a person who has been entitled to Social Security disability benefits for at least 24 months. A Medicare card is mailed out about 3 months before the 25th month of disability benefits.

A person with amyotrophic lateral sclerosis (also known as Lou Gehrig's disease) will get a Medicare card about 4 weeks after qualifying for Medicare.

A person with end-stage renal disease, or ESRD, does not need to be receiving Social Security disability benefits to qualify for Medicare, and may still be working.

The Centers for Medicare and Medicaid Services (CMS) administers Medicare, but the Social Security Administration (SSA) is responsible for enrolling most people in Medicare. The Railroad Retirement board is responsible for enrolling railroad retirees. For questions about Medicare enrollment, or to apply for Medicare benefits, call SSA at 1-800-772-1213

9. After people enroll in Medicare, how do they get their benefits?

People must decide how to get their Medicare benefits. They can choose Original Medicare, one of the Medicare Advantage Plans, or other Medicare health plans. If a person is receiving Social Security retirement benefits and does nothing when first eligible for Medicare, he or she will automatically be enrolled in Original Medicare.

10. What are some health care costs NOT covered by Medicare?

Medicare doesn't cover everything. For example, Medicare doesn't cover cosmetic surgery, health care you get while traveling outside of the United States (except in limited cases), hearing aids, most hearing exams, most eyeglasses, most dental care and dentures, and more. It also does not cover long-term care (except for skilled nursing care services that are needed daily on a short-term basis after a 3-day qualifying hospital stay). Some of these services may be covered by a Medicare Advantage Plan, such as an HMO (health maintenance organization) or PPO (preferred provider organization). A Medicare supplement can help with expenses not fully paid by Medicare.

11. What is Medigap?

People who choose Original Medicare may wish to consider Medigap, a type of Medicare supplement insurance. Medigap policies are sold by private insurance companies to fill gaps in Original Medicare Plan coverage, such as out-of-pocket costs for Medicare co-insurance and deductibles, or for services not covered by Medicare. A Medigap policy only works with Original Medicare. A person who joins a Medicare Advantage Plan generally doesn't need (and can't use) a Medigap policy.

12. What is the difference between Medicare and Medicaid?

Some people think that Medicare and Medicaid are the same. Actually, they are two different programs. Medicaid is a state-run program that provides hospital and medical coverage for people with low income and little or no resources. Each state has its own rules about who is eligible and what is covered under Medicaid. Some people qualify for both Medicare and Medicaid.

13. How does the Medicare PACE program help older adults?

PACE (Programs of All-Inclusive Care for the Elderly) combines medical, social, and long-term care services, and prescription drug coverage for frail, elderly people who get health care in the community.

To qualify for PACE, people must be at least age 55, live in the PACE service area, meet their state's standard for nursing home level care, and be able to live safely in a community setting at the time of enrollment.

Other MedicalCenter.com

Publications

The Key Facts on Arthritis

The Key Facts on Breast Cancer

All Titles Can Be Found at

www.Amazon.com

www.MedicalCenter.com